I0455753

Organic Makeup
Tips How to Make and Use Beautiful Homemade Makeup

All photos used in this book, including the cover photo were made available under a Attribution-NonCommercial-ShareAlike 2.0 Generic and sourced from Flickr

Copyright 2016 by the publisher - All rights reserved.

This document is geared towards providing exact and reliable information in regards to the topic and issue covered. The publication is sold with the idea that the publisher is not required to render accounting, officially permitted, or otherwise, qualified services. If advice is necessary, legal or professional, a practiced individual in the profession should be ordered.

- From a Declaration of Principles which was accepted and approved equally by a Committee of the American Bar Association and a Committee of Publishers and Associations.

In no way is it legal to reproduce, duplicate, or transmit any part of this document in either electronic means or in printed format. Recording of this publication is strictly prohibited and any storage of this document is not allowed unless with written permission from the publisher. All rights reserved.

The information provided herein is stated to be truthful and consistent, in that any liability, in terms of inattention or otherwise, by any usage or abuse of any policies, processes, or directions contained within is the solitary and utter responsibility of the recipient reader. Under no circumstances will any legal responsibility or blame be held against the publisher for any reparation, damages, or monetary loss due to the information herein, either directly or indirectly.

Respective authors own all copyrights not held by the publisher.

The information herein is offered for informational purposes solely, and is universal as so. The presentation of the information is without contract or any type of guarantee assurance.

The trademarks that are used are without any consent, and the publication of the trademark is without permission or backing by the trademark owner. All trademarks and brands within this book are for clarifying purposes only and are the owned by the owners themselves, not affiliated with this document.

Table of content

Introduction

It was not long ago when a compilation of designer and branded make up were announced to be dangerous to the health and had cancerous elements. And to think these lipsticks, eye shadows, blush powders and compact powders are super expensive ($20 for a lipstick, at the least). This is among the top reasons why makeup manufacturers have spent countless millions to re-study what went wrong with their chemicals and decided to go all natural.

Why women use makeup.

An online poll of about 3000 women said that they feel very confident leaving the house with makeup on (68%). About 1500 women or half of the respondents said that they wear makeup always. 41% said that they will not ever leave home without it on. A good 20% of the women in the poll admitted to wearing makeup in bed and applying lip gloss and mascara upon waking up in the morning. Well, whatever the real reason is, makeup makes the woman feel better inside and look really beautiful outside.

Some women are not blessed to have flawless skin. While some do not need to add a thick layer of foundation and lipstick, some have to cover up their blemishes, acne, pimple and other facial impurities. This is another reason why makeup is essential for some women to make their face seem flawless. This goes back to the original answer of feeling confident.

Mineral or all natural makeup is a better alternative.

It has been proven that non-mineral cosmetics can speed up the aging process and make the skin lose its elasticity. It may look good on the person wearing it but non-mineral makeup can also contribute to, at the most, cancer. You do not want this. The 20% of women in the poll wear makeup even while asleep and if they only knew they would not like it either. This is dangerous and harmful to the health. In the long run, it is not beauty anymore. It is deadly.

It is called mineral and all natural makeup because the color pigments in the makeup are composed of minerals. Just like the olden people thousands of years ago, they have the most radiant skin all because their makeup was extracted from natural substances.

All natural makeup is safe to use and even if you have it on overnight, you will have no problems with your skin and your health. Using mineral, all natural makeup is really nice and you will notice that the colors do not fade away easily. You will look more beautiful with all natural makeup powder, blush, lipstick and eye shadow. And all the solace comes when you decide to make the organic makeup all by yourself.

Chapter 1 – Overview Of Makeups

Once upon a time.... There existed some eras when beauty was the sphere for only girls. But those times have passed away. Now everyone seeks for beauty, be it a girl or a guy. While using rising demand of looking beautiful and garner a person's vision of most, the beauty industry reached its apex, now even nearby girl wish to appear to be her favorite Hollywood star!!

Due to these, the requirement for beauty items is increasing over the years. Subsequently, the rates of that merchandise are also increasing. If you're not careful, expensive beauty items can bite into their profits. It truly is worth taking into consideration the preparation and support what is required come up with a wise selection. But at the same time, it's correct there are many cosmetics of fine brands that may be a bit costly but could give your skin finest texture!

Products for natural skin care, hair care products, cosmetics, bath and body products, perfumes, body treatments, sun protection and self-tanning products, anti-aging and anti-wrinkle merchandise is most often used beauty products. These bath and body goods are accessible for both women and men, are lots of amongst options pocket-friendly.

However there are millions of means of you saving your bucks, the top practical method to limit the exact amount you commit to beauty products should be to go for homemade products. They allow these products by purchasing the specified ingredients and follow the instructions for sale. Also, the merchandise is from uncomfortable side effects that some store products at all. These unwanted side effects tend to be attributable to chemicals which are included with them to make sure they are more inviting and robust. Home-made beauty items all together will probably be much cheaper when compared with store-bought.

There are numerous techniques for making bath and body products that fit your financial budget. Purchasing the products on sale prices is a wonderful idea. You can also buy many of them in the case they are offered at good discounts. Do not always go with branded products. Sometimes you will realize that skin care products are almost the same quality however cheaper or expensive they are. Therefore, it is far better to acquire these products to save a lot of money. It's best to select skin care products that are reasonably priced. A high-end beauty product is possibly not excellent.

An alternate way to reduce costs is to find only products after walking around to identify the best favorable prices. Some stores offer several free samples. Cash back guarantees can also be given when the customer is not content with the product. So, be beautiful, go with great makeup that you can comfortably make at your home. Never achieving this by burning your pocket....

The Kit

You may already have things such as eyeliner, lipstick, and eye shadow but here are some things that you need to make sure you aren't missing. These items will allow you to touch yourself up when out on a date.

A vanity mirror, which is a small mirror, is something that you should have on hand. This is a great idea for checking yourself over privately since makeup and other hair disasters are quite common when you are in a rush. Trying to look at yourself in a window or reflection in a spoon won't be as good as it can be if you had a tiny mirror to look in to.

Skin balm is another must have in your travel makeup kit. A simple scrape of the face would be easily fixed with this balm. If you have no problem with petroleum jelly then you shouldn't have a problem. Rashes and hives are common with petroleum based products. It would be a disaster if your blemish became a hundred times worse. Body balm can also be used on the lips to make them look nicer and it also destroys bacteria that may be lurking.

Get natural looking rosy cheeks by using a cheek tint readily available in your makeup kit. You will always look like you've been in something romantic without looking overly made up. It will keep you looking glowing, but it will also lighten your mood knowing that you look good. Mix it with on a well-moisturized face to achieve that rosy glow.

Your kit should also include some mineral based powders. To prevent a shiny looking face you can use these powders to tone it down to a more natural looking tone. Mineral makeups are good for your skin so that is just another reason to use them. Mineral powders also work well with sensitive skin types.

Chapter 2 – Types Of Skins

It can be overwhelming to determine what the right skin care product is for you. We all have skin types that are as different as we are but knowing these and what this means can help you to get a plan and recipe that is just right for you. Knowing your skin type will not only make your efforts more effective but replenish the actual needs of your body, allowing it to respond in a completely organic way. Building this type of relationship with your skin will make sure that it will stay clean, vibrant, and healthy.

Before this type of partnership can be built, it is important to know what classifies as a skin type. The three major classifications are built upon these characteristics: dry, normal, or oily. Although these words may seem very plain, understanding their meaning allows for you to regain control of your skin care. To find out which type your skin is you can use a mirror and examine your face (forehead, nose, and chin) for these qualities: elasticity, complexion, and pore and blemish visibility.

For example, if your complexion is taught, having little elasticity, and bearing little to no blemishes, your skin would easily qualify for a dry skin type. However, if your skin is loose, bears a full or oily complexion, and contains many blemishes your skin would qualify as an oily skin type. A face that seems to show a balanced result is called normal.

An important factor to think about while evaluating your skin is any other outside factors that may affect your skin's condition. Genetics, medication, or the chemicals and temperatures it's exposed to may play an important role in properly evaluating your skin. Determining these will allow you to make informed decisions that may lead to a much more accurate skin type analysis. Some skin conditions that affect skin type may require a doctor, such as a dermatologist to properly restore or balance your body's current skin quality and condition. After these important stages are accomplished it is now possible to accurately address your unique skin condition.

Wrinkles

While the presence wrinkles are mostly the result of genetics and the natural aging process, they are also caused by smoking, excess sun exposure, dehydration, and repetitive facial expressions such as smiling, frowning, or squinting.

Dull skin

A dull complexion can appear drab in color, tired, and stressed. Dull skin can be caused by lack of proper cleansing, inadequate sleep, dehydration, poor circulation, and a poor diet consisting of processed foods. Exfoliation helps in removal of lifeless skin cells that get in the way of the healthy glowing skin.

Dry Skin

Dry skin is characterized by small pores, along with a consistent lack of moisture than leads to an uncomfortable tight feeling. Dry skin is particularly prone to fine lines, wrinkles, and broken capillaries.

Oily Skin

Oily skin is prone to mild and severe acne, blackheads, whiteheads, and enlarged pores. Due to excess moisture, dry skin is less likely to become prematurely wrinkled.

Acne-Prone Skin

Skin that is prone to acne can be easily irritated by commercial solutions designed to treat the problem, as these treatments tend to strip the skin of its natural protective oils. The common factors associated with acne are genetics, excess oil production, and a diet high in sugar, wheat, and dairy.

Sensitive Skin

Sensitive skin can affect both dry and oily skin types. It is easily irritated by harsh skin products that are loaded with chemical additives. Dry sensitive skin is dry and fragile, and can easily become irritated by environmental conditions and certain skin products. When overly washed, the pores of oily sensitive skin can release an over-production of sebum.

Mature Skin

Mature skin is known for its lack of elasticity, compared to younger skin. It tends to be looser, drier, and duller, due to a decrease in sebum production. Mature skin can appear to be heavily lined, thin, and taut.

Combination Skin

Most people have combination skin, with dryness around the cheeks and eyes, and excess oil production on the forehead, nose, and chin. This type of skin is generally treated by specific area, for best results.

Selecting your Makeup

Makeups have become an essential part of a beauty regime. Even though makeups should not be utilized on a day to day basis, most skin experts suggest that makeups are safe to utilize weekly or even twice a week. Removing dead skin cells and exfoliating the skin is important because it promotes healthy growth and also increases the suppleness of the body.

Keeping this in mind, it is essential to take into account the type of skin you have. Not all makeups are suited for every skin type because each has specific characteristics and reactions that have to be taken care of. Even though a lot of the basic ingredients in most makeups are the same, there are some substances whose efficacy varies from skin to skin.

Chapter 3 – The Rules

There are literally thousands of makeup and beauty products out there on the market. There are also a lot of homemade makeup and beauty recipes. Below are some makeup and beauty warnings to watch out for when applying makeup or using beauty products.

1. Do an allergy test. Test out your makeup and beauty products first before you use them. This will teach you whether or not you will have an allergic reaction to the product before it spreads to the rest of your body.

2. Don't use a foundation that changes color. Foundation shouldn't change color after you've applied it. If you notice either your foundation or concealer changing color or looking more orange, throw it away.

3. Stay away from cheap makeup. Cheap makeup will never make you look your best, and on many occasions will actually make you look worse. Stick to high-quality makeup that will help you look your best.

4. Avoid wearing makeup when you are going to the gym or going on a long, intense run. Makeup can cause your pore to clog, which can eventually cause some issues for your skin. It's much better to wash off your makeup before working out, and then freshening it up afterward.

5. Look for any threatening foundation lines on your face. Foundation and concealers, if not blended properly, can have issues with looking mask-like. Blend your foundation and pay attention near your jaw and chin to make sure your face looks as natural as possible.

6. Don't let family or friends borrow your makeup. This is especially true for eyeliners and mascara. This is a quick way to spread eye infections.

7. Don't avoid sunscreen. Sunscreen is very helpful with protecting your skin from harmful UV rays. A lot of sunscreens is automatically put in sunscreen, but if your foundation does not be sure to apply it on your face before putting on the rest of your makeup.

Makeup - Dos And Don'ts

Tip 1. Do not use makeup on damaged or broken skin.

Tip 2. Do not use glass containers in the bathroom so they don't slip and break, use plastic containers instead.

Tip 3. Do not allow water to get in your makeup as it will cause the growth of mold. Store in air-tight jars in a cool, dry place.

Tip 4. Discard makeups with rancid smells or visible signs of molds.

Chapter 4 – Prepare Your Makeup

Ever been turned back by the massive amount of chemicals found on the back of so many cosmetic products, including the makeups you use so often? Many people have been. With products all across the board becoming more and more expensive, a great place to start saving money is with things you use often. Homemade makeups are incredibly easy to make and can be made quickly with very common ingredients from the kitchen.

Some oils are very useful. Each oil listed below has unique benefits and all work well. Try using several of them until you find the combination of ingredients that works best for you and your skin.

Olive Oil

Olive oil has an extensive history of versatility. Dating back to 400 B.C., it was used not only in food applications but also in skin care as a moisturizer and perfume. Its chemical composition is similar to oils in our skin making it easily absorbed and a great natural moisturizer. It is rich in antioxidants and aids in our skins' production of collagen and elastin. It can be used as a makeup remover as well, though may not break down some cosmetics as well as store bought makeup removers.

Sunflower Oil

Sunflower oil has many health benefits such as reducing the risk of cardiovascular disease, arthritis prevention and maintaining a healthy nervous system. Similar to olive oil, it is rich in antioxidants and Vitamin E, which helps cells retain water and therefore stay moisturized.

Castor Oil

When you think of castor oil, you might think of motor oil. Castor oil is in fact extremely versatile and is used in products ranging from lipstick, plastics, brake fluid to shampoo. The FDA has deemed it "generally safe and effective," as it is safe to consume in small quantities as a laxative. In skin care applications, castor oil is used to treat skin disorders and infections and its molecular mass is small enough to penetrate the epidermis, making it an effective moisturizer. For these reasons, castor oil can be safely used as a base to your homemade makeup.

Making Your Own Mascara

If you've got problems with spending too much money on mascara, or having a hard time finding nontoxic ones, making your own homemade mascara recipe could be a solution for you. You basically just mix a pigment color (powdered eye shadow) of your choice, with Aloe Vera gel.

You just use Aloe Vera gel and makeup pigments and mix them together 50/50 in whatever amount of mascara that you want to make. If you want to make an ounce, then you would use 1/2 ounce of gel, and 1/2 ounce of pigment.

The key is to find inexpensive ingredients to make your own mascara. Powdered eye shadow can be pretty expensive right now, especially because mineral make-up is all the trend right now.

The Aloe Vera gel should be even easier to buy in bulk, because it's really not that popular of a product in terms of trends.

Homemade Lavender lip balm.

Ingredients:

- 4 tablespoons olive oil or almond.

- 1 tablespoon honey.

- 1 tablespoon Beeswax pearls.

- 7 drops Lavender oil.

- Cocoa powder.

If you would like some color, you will also need a teaspoon of colored lipstick preferably natural.

Procedure.

Start by melting the beeswax and honey in a bowl that is made of stainless steel. Make sure that you use low heat and keep stirring until you have both of the ingredients well melted, remove from the heat and add the essential oil of your choice and throw in the colored lipstick the vitamin E and the cocoa powder if you choose to add this and lastly, you can set the concoction in an ice water pan and then continue whisking as you add the honey. After it has mixed well, you can then place the mixture in your lip balm container and let is solidify for the next three hours after which it is ready to use.

Coco Rosey.

This is one of those lip balm recipes that have that soothing effect to your lips. It is among those lip balms that quickly become a companion at all times.

Ingredients:

- Dried rosebuds

- 2 tablespoons Coconut oil

- 1 tablespoon coconut butter

- Vitamin E

- 3 drops Essential oil (rose oil)

Procedure.

Start by melting the coconut oil and as usual you should make sure that you use a stainless steel on very low heat. After it has melted add in the roses or whichever other dried flower that you opted for and keep stirring. Let it steep for another hour still on low heat then strain into a bowl. Clean out the original container and place it back in the heat. Place the oil you have just strained back into the original container and while still heating, add the essential oil and Vitamin E and keep stirring then remove from the fire and place the mixture in a small skillet and allow to solidify.

Minty Chocolate lip balm.

This lip balm has two of the things that most of the women fall in love with. These are a chocolaty taste and a minty breath. It can't get better than that.

Ingredients:

- 1 tablespoon Cocoa butter.
- 1 tablespoon Honey.
- 1 tablespoon Shea butter.
- 1 tablespoon Grated beeswax.
- 1/8 cup Coconut oil
- 1 tablespoon Cocoa powder.
- 3 drops Peppermint
- 1/8 cup vitamin oil.

Procedure.

Start with the coconut oil, Shea and the cocoa butter and place them in an appropriate container and heat under low heat for about 20 minutes while at the same stirring though occasionally. Stir in the beeswax and let it to completely melt. Kill the heat. Stir in the remaining ingredients to obtain a uniform mixture. Store in a smaller glass container.

The best thing is about homemade lip balm is not the fact that it is cheaper and easy to make but it lets you use ingredients that you are confident about and those that you're confident will be of help.

Chapter 5 – Hair And Makeup

One of the defining trait and characteristics of mammals are their hair. Some mammals cover their whole body with hairs, others have hairs In specific regions of the body. In case of humans they have the most organized and well-developed structure in all mammals.. In addition to skin, hairs protruding from the dermal layer of skin also form a protective covering over the body. Hairs have a number of biological uses and act as an essential part of human body.Hairs on the heads protect us from the UV (ultraviolet) rays coming from the sun and from the debris. Hairs near the eyebrow region help in deflecting back the harmful debris. Likewise, hairs act as a major protection against the excessive heat. The functions of hairs for the external protection are numerous. Hairs inside help the body to maintain balance and posture. Our orientation with respect to gravity is solely controlled by those hairs. Despite their biological importance hairs play a significant role in making up and grooming a person's personality.

Importance of Dressing up:

In social gatherings and functions people tend to dress up so that they look appeal-able. In acquiring that noticeable appearance people often women wear makeup and style their hairs in a way that they look attracting and gorgeous. Hairs act as a reflection of our personalities. They act as our identity in personal and social life. Many of the men and women are of the view that "A bad hair day equals to Bad day". Hairstyle of a person more often tells the psyche and self-esteem of the person. A popular hairstyle with the right makeup is appealable and attracting to people. Wearing makeup is perhaps the best hobby of women.

Choosing right makeup over the dressing and styling the most suitable hairs for an occasion is the first approach of every woman.

Chapter 6 – Applying The Makeup

If you apply Makeup in the correct manner, you will improve your features and have a wonderful look. You need to know how to use them for you to get the full benefits and avoid the artificial ones.

Procedural tips

Cleanse Your Face Carefully. You may start by going to the bathroom. Wet your body in the shower from head to toe.

Feet should be dealt with first then the other parts to follow..

Remove rough spots and calluses on your face using a soft material. If you have a very rough face, add a cup of milk to a basin of warm water, stir and soak your face using a soft towel for 30 minutes before entering the shower.

Scrub your face gently. Pay attention to your mouth and eyes but you must use an exfoliating product meant for the face because it is gentle than those made for the body.

Remember your hands; they should look and feel soft too.

Rinse your body using lukewarm water

Step out of the shower

The previous steps ensured that your skin is clean and good for the application of the makeup. Basically you need to cleanse your skin, tone it and then moisturize it. You begin by applying cream or cleansing milk to your forehead, cheekbones and nose. With a clean cotton wool gently clean your face in small circular movements. Rinse your face with cold water.

The next step is shaping your eyebrows. Do away with any stray hairs using a pair of tweezers. Pluck any excess hairs towards the direction it is growing.

Use the makeup alongside a sunscreen and use your fingertips or a sponge to apply it outwardly to get a smooth and even toning. The more natural the makeup is, the better. Apply sunscreen if you are going out in the sun. You do not want the fresh skin to be damaged by the sun especially since it may be slightly irritated. Lightly cover your cheeks, forehead and chin regions. Start applying from the center as you go outwards to jaw-line to ensure that the makeup has a smooth finish.

Add color to the makeup. For example, use the cream for dry skins and powder eye shadow on oily skin.

Apply a loose powder to do away with any excessive shine which will enable the makeup to stay longer. Ensure that you use a face powder that matches with your natural skin complexity. Transparent ones are the best. Use a face powder brush to evenly distribute the powder working from the inside as you head outwards.

Apply a blusher using a brush.

Remember the eye shadow? Dot the right shade of concealer under your eye.

Evenly apply an eye base to firmly hold the eye shadow on the eyelid for long.

Define your lips by utilizing a lip liner and ensure that there is no bleeding out of the lipstick. Blend with a brush and apply gloss if need be.

Ensure you use facial moisturizers and body lotions that contain alpha or beta hydroxy acids because they help in removing dead skin cells.

Extra Tips:

Preserve the smoothness and avoid breakouts by using a non-comedogenic moisturizer.

Don't apply the makeup too hard to your face, this can cause damage to and hurt your skin. Do not exfoliate if you have an open wound or cut or if you are sunburned. Although a variety of makeups are available on the market these days. They are filled with addictive and preservatives that could harm your skin in the long run. It is advisable to be cautious of what we absorb into our skin. It is unrealistic to eat organic foods and then introduce chemicals into our bodies through our skin. The solution to a wonderful skin is in your kitchen, not the store!

Chapter 7 – Homemade Facials

Essential skin care elements have not changed. Get plenty of sleep, keep your skin hydrated with a good moisturizer, and give yourself a facial once a week.

While facials or beauty masks are often associated with pampering for the relief, it does not need to be expensive and can be done quickly and easily from home. A weekly facial helps revitalize the skin, removing dead skin cells, deep cleansing pores and stimulating circulation.

While you can certainly purchase either clay or gel beauty masks, you might find them too harsh on sensitive skin. Besides, there's really no need when you can find the best skin care solutions in your local grocery store or supermarket.

Some products are very good to be used for your face and neck include, oatmeal, bananas, avocados, yogurt or even milk. Mixing a little milk with oatmeal, for example, is a fantastic remedy for dry, tired skin.

Before applying your mask, thoroughly clean your skin, removing all traces of dirt and makeup. Rinse your face with warm to hot water to help open your pores and allow the mask to penetrate. Coat your face and neck with a thick layer of your mask, using circular motions to help stimulate circulation. Be careful to avoid the fragile skin around the eyes. Leave the mask on for about twenty minutes to thirty minutes.

While your mask is working, you may wish to lie back and relax with soothing sounds or your favorite music. A couple of cooled teabags or cucumber slices are good for covering your eyes while you rest. This will alleviate any puffiness and replenish lost moisture to the sensitive eye area.

When you are done, rinse your face and neck with tepid water to remove all traces of the mask. Avoid rubbing too hard, keeping the use of facecloths or buffs to a minimum. Once the mask has been cleaned away, splash cold water on your face several times to close the pores. Follow up with your favorite toner (if desired) and of course, moisturizer.

A weekly homemade facial will keep your skin in top form, healthy, smooth, well hydrated and revitalized...

Conclusion

The art of applying makeup is one that has to be practiced. Most women make two mistakes when it comes to applying makeup; the first one is to use too much and the second one is to use the wrong shades and colors. Both can make you look artificial and caked up and unattractive. The right way to use makeup is in moderate amounts so that you look radiant and natural.

If you follow these simple steps, applying makeup will not seem like a chore but an enjoyable experience to help you look your best.

Whatever your choice is when making your own homemade makeup, you're rest assured you are saving money and are using perfectly safe and healthy ingredients on your skin. Best of luck in your search for the combination that works best for you!

FREE Bonus Reminder

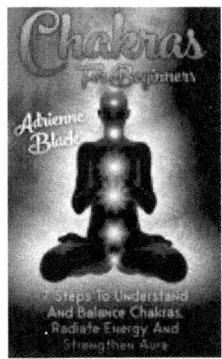

If you have not grabbed it yet, please go ahead and download your special bonus E book *"Chakras for Beginners. 7 Steps To Understand And Balance Chakras, Radiate Energy, And Strengthen Aura"*.

Simply Click the Button Below

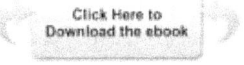

OR Go to This Page

http://lifehacksworld.com/free

BONUS #2: More Free & Discounted Books & Products

Do you want to receive more Free/Discounted Books or Products?

We have a mailing list where we send out our new Books or Products when they go free or with a discount on Amazon. Click on the link below to sign up for Free & Discount Book & Product Promotions.

=> **Sign Up for Free & Discount Book & Product Promotions** <=

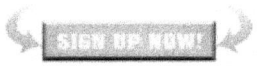

OR Go to this URL

http://zbit.ly/1WBb1Ek

www.ingramcontent.com/pod-product-compliance
Lightning Source LLC
Chambersburg PA
CBHW072022290526
45787CB00013B/1758